Luxurious Bath Bombs
40 Bath Bomb Recipes

Jenny De Luca

CONTENTS

ACKNOWLEDGMENTS

Any copyrights and trademarks mentioned within this book are fully acknowledged.

As someone who has bought this book on Amazon, you are entitled to a free download of the Kindle version. This will enable you to get the full-color book in electronic format. Unfortunately, I have to publish these books in black and white in order to make them affordable due to the high cost of color printing. Please download this from Amazon; you can read it on a Kindle, or any tablet, cell phone or computer with the free Kindle Reader installed from your app store.

Why Make and Use Bath Bombs?

Making your own bath bombs is a fun hobby and they make great gifts that people love to receive. Who knows, perhaps you will enjoy it so much you will turn it into a business, selling your bath bombs and beauty products at craft fairs, online or even opening your own store. After all, the global franchise Lush was started by someone making their own beauty products at home and now look at it, it's a successful global franchise!

One of the really big advantages of making your own bath bombs is that you can tailor the ingredients to your specific needs. If you have an allergy to a particular substance or you like a particular oil, then you can make your bath bombs using those. This saves both time and money from trying to find them at the shops, which can be hard if you like the more unusual ingredients or wish to avoid certain ingredients.

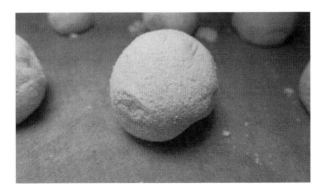

Making your own bath bombs isn't particularly difficult to do, as you will find out, and you can make them as complex or as simple as you want.

It is up to you exactly how much effort you put in to them, with the possibilities limited only by your imagination! Once you understand the basic recipe, you can make all sorts of variations on the theme and be incredibly creative in what you produce.

One ingredient though that you should avoid is borax and you will occasionally see this mentioned as an ingredient in some recipes. It should be avoided as it is used as ant poison, is toxic and considered carcinogenic! As this chemical is absorbed through the skin, it is one ingredient that is important to avoid.

Corn flour is recommended in some recipes, including some in this book because it makes your skin feel nice. However, if you suffer from yeast infections or candida, you should avoid recipes that contain this ingredient or omit it from the recipe as it will feed the infections and potential make them worse.

Most of the other ingredients that you will use in making bath bombs are easy to get hold of locally. Some ingredients may need buying online to get the best prices and large enough quantities for what you are planning on making. If you are buying in bulk, then online is usually far cheaper, which is important if you are aiming to produce a profit from your efforts.

When you start making bath bombs, you will realize that it is a lot of fun and very rewarding, not just from enjoying laying in the bath and relaxing with your own creation, but also by making them as gifts for people you know. They are a simple gift and do not have to cost the earth, but are very meaningful because people will know you have made them by hand and taken the time to produce something lovely for them. It will be very much appreciated, and you never know … you may be getting orders from your friends and family soon! I often give home-made beauty products as presents to my friends and they are always well received, particularly when I go to the effort to present them nicely.

Enjoy making bath bombs and most of all enjoy experimenting with oils and other ingredients to make the most wonderful sensory experiences for the bath. With herbs, petals, glitter and other ingredients you can make some incredibly creative recipes. Some people even hide little plastic toys in their bath bombs if they are making them for children. There are lots and lots of possibilities and this book will introduce you to many of them, so you can let your imagination run wild as you have fun producing your own bath bombs at home.

SHAPING AND MOLDING YOUR BATH BOMBS

When you buy bath bombs in the stores you will see they are often made in elaborate shapes and you wonder how it is done. However, don't worry, I'll explain how you can make some great looking bath bombs and it is much easier than you may have thought!

Firstly, you do not need any special equipment to shape your bath bombs. You can shape them into the standard ball shape, which is great for beginners whilst you are getting used to the process or you can mold them into other shapes by hand if you are feeling artistic. Although you can roughly shape them by hand into the traditional ball, most people will use molds as it is easier to get a consistent size and shape, as well as hold the balls together.

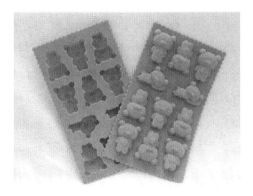

If you want to make things more interesting then you can buy special bath bomb molds, but these are not exactly cheap and can be quite limited in the available designs. What you can do instead is buy candy, jello or candle molds and use those to shape your bath bombs! Simple isn't it and it is a great way to get superb looking bath bombs at a good price. Silcone molds are by far the best because it is easier to get your bath bombs out without breaking them.

Some of the best silicone molds I have found are from www.amazon.com/shops/baileyinc who produce molds such as those shown above.

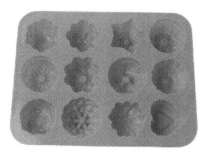

Craft stores will have a wide variety of different molds that you can use, though there are many improvisations possible. What about cutting a tennis ball in half to make a mold for a round bath bomb? What about using a muffin tray or an ice cube tray or even some shot glasses? If you have a look around your kitchen right now you can probably find a number of things that you can use as molds for your bath bombs.

You need to make sure that whatever you use for a mold is clean, dry and is not going to leave any debris on your bath bomb as that will spoil it. When shaping your bath bombs, you will find that smaller bath bombs are much easier to make than larger ones as the larger bombs are more likely to crumble, while the smaller ones are much more robust. This is because it takes longer and is harder for the large bath bombs to dry evenly, while the smaller ones dry quicker. Inconsistent drying is a common cause of crumbly bath bombs.

There are a lot of different types of molds you can use, and this is a great opportunity for you to be creative and either create something for a holiday season or to appeal to a particular person or market. The candy or jello molds are not expensive and will cost you no more than a few bucks with the vast majority being under ten dollars. You can order them online or buy them from a local cookware store, though often you can find the simpler molds in grocery stores too.

Using molds made of silicone is by far the best because it is much easier to keep them clean and to get your bath bombs out of the mold without breaking them. Solid molds made from metal or hard plastic are much harder to get the bombs out without damaging them. Just ensure that the bath bombs have had plenty of drying time before you try to remove them as removing them to early will lead to them crumbling.

Storing Your Bath Bombs

Bath bombs are designed to dissolve in water, so it is very important they are stored properly because otherwise they will dissolve and melt if they get damp. You certainly don't want your hard work melting away and to be wasted. Correct storage is very important and so let's cover some of the best ways to store your bath bombs, so they last a good few weeks, if not several months.

Ideally you want to keep your bath bombs in a moisture free environment. You can package them in zip lock bags, though squeeze out all the air first as that will help prevent the bath bombs absorbing moisture. Some people will shrink wrap their bath bombs in plastic, which is probably one of the best ways to store your bath bombs, though obviously you have the cost of the shrink wrap equipment. Plastic wrap will also work well as a method for storing your bath bombs. A vacuum sealer is another great way to store your bath bombs. Package each one separately and vacuum pack each one. Sucking the air out ensures no moisture remains and the bath bomb remains good for much longer.

Your bath bombs need to be stored in a cool, dark, dry place which will help prevent them from melting. Some people will store them in the refrigerator, but other people will store them in the back of a cupboard or drawer. Just be careful they don't get damaged though as they are still quite fragile. Saying that, if they do get damaged you can still put them in the bath, they just don't look the same.

Many people store their bath bombs in plastic or metal containers as these are usually air tight. If you can get hold of packets of silica gel, which can be found in any electrical products you buy or bought online, then these are worth putting in the containers to absorb any moisture.

To be fair, most people will use their bath bombs pretty quickly, so they aren't going to require storing for too long, but you can usually store one for a few weeks and up to several months in the right conditions!

Presenting Your Bath Bombs

If you are planning on giving your bath bombs as gifts or selling them, then you need to present them nicely. Here is an opportunity for you to use your imagination and really be creative. If you are selling them, then professional packaging is an absolute must to be taken seriously and command a good price.

When you visit a craft store you will find squares of thick plastic wrap which are typically used to wrap soap. These are great to wrap around your bath bombs, usually being just the right size and can be tied with some colored ribbon so they look more attractive.

With smaller bath bombs you can present them in small boxes or even glass tumblers or jars as they will look good. You can still cover them with plastic to keep the moisture out and decorate the jars as you want.

Shrink wrapping your bath bombs can make them look very professional, though a shrink wrap machine is necessary, but they can be bought for under $50 for a cheap one, though the better machines are more expensive. However, this can be a way to make your bath bombs look great and stop the moisture getting to them, which will be important if you are selling them.

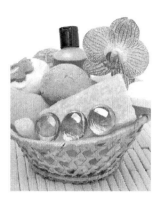

Of course, you can present your bath bombs in baskets (available from craft stores) and then wrapped in plastic, tied with ribbon and perhaps filled with other home-made or natural products plus fillers such as petals, sea shells and so on.

Another alternative is to use presentation boxes, again available from a craft store, though these are generally not see through, so you don't get the "wow factor" from people seeing your home-made products.

At the end of the day a walk around a large craft store is going to fill your head full of ideas and empty your bank account. You will see plenty of different ways to present your bath bombs. Have a look around your local craft stores and get some ideas. What you are planning on doing with your bath bombs will influence how you present them. If you are making them for home use, then the presentation is not as important. However, if you are planning to give the bath bombs as gifts or sell them, then presentation becomes much more important.

When selling your bath bombs, look at how those that are sold are packaged. Look around stores and at craft markets. Many people sell the bath bombs loose and put them in paper bags when sold. This does work and the advantage of this is that people can smell and touch the bath bombs before purchasing. However, the disadvantage is that they can touch the bath bombs and potentially damage your stock.

If you are selling your bath bombs, you can plastic wrap them all, but leave just one of each variety unwrapped or loosely wrapped so that people can smell and appreciate the quality of your product. Professional, quality packaging can mean people will pay a premium price and it protects their purchase from damage.

Even packaging your bath bombs for home use can help protect them and allow them to store well. The other advantage if you package them is that if you are ever caught short on a birthday present, you have some bath bombs in stock!

Packaging isn't essential unless you are selling or gifting your bath bombs. It's a fun part of making them and gives you another opportunity to express your creativity.

HOW TO MAKE BUBBLE BARS

Bubble bars are great in the bath because they give you the relaxed feeling that you get from bubble bath with a much thicker foam and stronger smell. The bubble bars foam and dissolve when placed under running water. These can be spiced and fragranced in any way you want, we'll talk more about that shortly. You can mold them anyway you want or just use a standard bread loaf tin (available from cook shops and supermarkets) and cut the bars into slices.

Ingredients:
- 1 cup baking sofa
- 1 cup sodium lauryl sulfoacetate
- 2ml essential oil (of your choice)
- 1 tablespoon cream of tartar
- Liquid glycerine
- Food coloring (optional)

Method:
1. Pour the baking soda into a glass bowl
2. If you want to make a bubble bar of a different color, then remove ¼ cup of baking soda, pour it into another bowl and add some food coloring, stirring well to combine before adding back to the original bowl
3. Add 2ml of an essential oil (or mixture of oils) to the mixture and stir well
4. Add a tablespoon of cream of tartar and whisk until thoroughly combined

5. Add in the sodium lauryl sulfoacetate powder (this creates the foaming appearance and is made from palm and coconut oil) and whisk well, ensuring it is well mixed

6. Add four or five drops of liquid glycerine and stir well

7. Sprinkle some baking soda into your mold and pour in the bubble bar liquid

8. Leave it to sit for around ten minutes so it begins to harden

9. Turn the mold over on to a piece of parchment paper and gently tap the bottom of the mold until the bar falls out. If it crumbly then put it back into the mold and add some more liquid glycerine, leave it a few more minutes and then turn it out again

10. Leave the bubble bar to solidify and then cut into slices and store in a cool, dry, dark place in a sealed container

These bubble bars are not hard to make and are a great addition to bath bombs if you are giving gifts but also a lovely gift to yourself for a luxurious bath! These benefit from being wrapped in greaseproof or baking paper, which helps to protect them. Clear, thick plastic sheets can also be used. Do not store these so they are directly touching each other as there is a risk that they will fuse together. These, like bath bombs, make an excellent gift and can be sold together with your bath bombs.

Basic Bath Bomb Recipe

There will be lots of bath bomb recipes coming up soon, but before you learn all of those let's just talk about the basic recipe for the bath bomb. Once you know this, you can vary and adjust the recipe as you see fit to create your own recipes and variations to suit your specific needs.

The basic recipe requires just three ingredients

1. 2 parts sodium bicarbonate (baking soda)
2. 1 part citric acid (powder)
3. A little bit of water

This is very easy to turn into a bath bomb; the basic process is as follows:

1. Mix the dry ingredients together

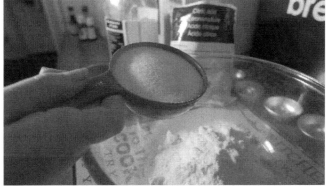

2. Spray in a little bit of water so the dry ingredients start to clump

together

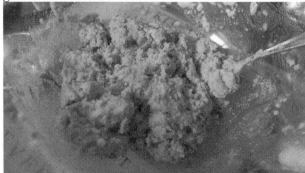

3. Press the mixture into the molds, leave for a short while to solidify and dry before removing from the mold
4. Leave to dry on a surface for a couple of days

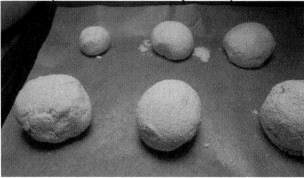

A good starting amount is 4oz of the baking soda and 2oz of citric acid, though you can make a little bit more and put it to one side in case you make the mixture too wet. Add the water a little bit at a time as it is very easy to make the mixture too wet and sticky, so it doesn't form proper bath bombs. The best way to do this is to use a spray bottle to spray water or witch hazel into the mixture. After a few sprays, stir the mixture and it should start to clump together and not crumble. If you squash the clumps of the mixture against the edge of your bowl with the back of a spoon you can easily tell if it is wet enough as it sticks to the bowl, but water does not leak out. If water does leak out when you press against the mixture, then you know that it is too wet and needs more of the dry mixture adding.

Getting the right consistency is probably the hardest part of making a bath bomb and there are a lot of things that affect this including using essential oils, adding petals or any other ingredients. Even the temperature in the room you are working in will influence the consistency, so you need to learn by trial and error, though I will try to explain as best I can.

The right consistency for a bath bomb is like perfect snow, i.e. it is powdery when you move it with a spoon yet push on it or squeeze it and it packs together. One good test for this is to squeeze a lump of the mixture in your hand then drop it back in the bowl. If it falls apart then you need more water, but if it stays mostly together the consistency is fine.

If the mixture is doughy and sticks to your fingers, then it is too wet, and you need to add more of the dry ingredients to loosen it up. Remember that if you are adding essential oils you will need less water. Sometimes you will hear a loud crackling or hissing sound from the mixture which also indicates it is too wet, though even when the consistency is fine you will usually hear a very faint hissing of the water reacting with the baking soda.

Your mixture is too dry if it slides through your fingers like sand, is crumbly, or when you clump it together it holds its shape before falling apart again. With the latter though you are very close to getting the right consistency. When you have the right consistency, it is easy for you to mold and shape the bath bombs, plus much easier for you to remove the bombs from the mold. If the consistency is wrong, add more water, a little at a time or add more dry mixture (with the 2/1 ratio of sodium bicarbonate to citric acid) a little at a time. By going slowly, you are more likely to get the consistency right and not have to spend a lot of your time adding more ingredients, so you end up with far too much mixture.

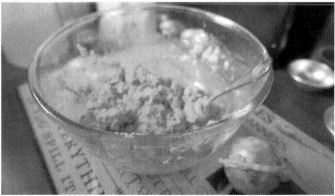

A bath bomb mixture in progress

With the right consistency the bath bombs will literally drop straight out of the mold without sticking to it. You can just wipe the mold clean and then use it again for more bath bombs! Do not leave your mixture sitting around before you mold it, i.e. make the mixture and mold it immediately because if you leave it, the water starts to evaporate off and the bath bombs end up cracking.

Because of the importance of getting the right consistency, it is better to make your bath bomb mixture in small batches rather than make a large amount which then sits around for ages before hardening in the bowl.

Molding is a bit of an art form and you will perfect it with practice, so just be patient with yourself when you start out. Remember that if a bath bomb does fall to pieces you can gather up the pieces and throw them in your bath, they will still work!

If you are using molds that are in halves then you spoon the mixture into one half then fill the other half before pushing them together, squeezing tightly for a little while so the two halves stick together. Remember once you have de-molded your bath bombs they need leaving on a clean, dry surface for a couple of hours, which allows them to solidify and fully dry out.

Coloring Bath Bombs

Coloring your bath bombs is very easy to do. Firstly, you need to use a coloring that is safe for use on humans. Most people will use food colorings as they are cheap, easy to get hold of and perfectly safe for you to use. There are other colorings available for cosmetic use, though many people report they do not give vibrant enough colors without using a lot of it.

The food coloring is added to the mixture whilst it is dry, before you add the water. Do not add it to the water and then spray it on the dry mixture because you will not get the same depth of color. The final result will have a very washed out color due to the dilution.

How many drops you use will depend on how deep you want the color to be and the quality of the coloring. Remember that the coloring reduces the amount of water required to reach the right consistency. There are limits to the amount of food coloring you can add to a bath bomb because the mixture can get too wet and then it won't stick together properly. This is why quality of coloring is so important. An alternative to food coloring is food grade mica powder, which can provide a more vibrant color.

You need to ensure the coloring is distributed evenly throughout your bath bomb otherwise you end up with a swirly pattern which, in some cases, can be pleasant but often not what the desired result. As you add the water the color will be distributed throughout the mixture as it is stirred.

You can buy powdered colorant from craft stores or online. These are great for bath bombs and gives you a much more even distribution of color. They cost more than food coloring, but is really good for strong, vibrant colors. You don't need a lot of coloring to get a good quality color. These types of coloring are great if you are regularly making bath bombs.

To make bath bombs with swirled colors or even layered colors will require a little bit more time, but can make for some superb looking bath bombs. Mix everything up as normal and then before you add the color and water, separate the mixture into separate bowls, one for each color.

Mix the color and the water in each of the bowls and then you can layer the mixture in the mold or you can mix the contents of the bowls together to create a swirl effect. Adding all the colors to one bowl doesn't get the same effect and you end up with patchy looking bath bombs or bombs that are a boring and unpleasant color. If you are using separate bowls, make sure that each mixture is the right consistency because otherwise you can end up with cracks in your bath bombs where one mixture is wetter than another and it dries unevenly.

Adding Grains, Petals and Herbs

These are a great addition to your bath bombs to give them a little something special. All sorts of different ingredients can be added to help benefit your skin, add texture, smell or just to make them look more interesting. While flower petals and herbs don't really do much for your skin, it does add to the luxury of the bath bomb and makes the bath look fantastic afterwards.

Oatmeal / Porridge Oats
These are a very popular additive to bath bombs as they are good at helping people who suffer from itchy skin. The oats make the water goey and soothing for the skin, but you do have to be careful not to add too much because your bath can end up like a bowl of porridge or it can clog the drain.

Clay
White clay makes for a good additive as it helps your bath bombs dry better and crack less. It does add a silky, smooth texture to the water, though it can be drying to your skin, so perhaps add some oils to compensate for that.

Aloe Powder

This is harder to find and is freeze dried aloe vera, which is incredibly good for your skin. You can often find 100x strength which is like bathing in pure aloe juice, though it doesn't have the same gel consistency that it has when it comes out of the plant. It is great for sunburn or anyone who suffers from skin irritations.

Milk or Yogurt Powder

You can use cow or goat milk powder, which is easily found at a health food store and is known to be soft and hydrating to your skin. It feels fantastic, though make sure you buy the full fat powder rather than a reduced fat version because it is the fat in the milk which gives the water the texture.

Lathering Agents

Using a lathering agent such as Sodium Laureth Sulfate will help make the bath bomb foam as it dissolves which can make for a very inviting looking bath!

Salts

Adding about a cup of salt such as Epsom, Sea or Dead Sea salts to your bath bomb can be really effective and relaxing. You may find it helpful to use some clay together with the salt in order to bind the bath bomb together properly as the salt crystals can weaken the bomb.

Butters

There are lots of different types of butters you can add to your bombs which will help your skin and make the water feel fantastic. There are many different varieties available including coconut, shea, cocoa, coffee, mango, aloe and more. Ensure you adjust the quantity of water in your mixture so you get the right consistency.

As you can see, making a bath bomb is just the start of the process, there are many other things you can do which will help make them much more interesting and inviting. If you are planning on selling or giving away your bath bombs, then the addition of these extra ingredients can command a premium price and make your products look more attractive.

TROUBLESHOOTING YOUR BATH BOMBS

Occasionally you will have problems with your bath bombs, but most of the time they are going to be just fine. In this section, you are going to learn some of the common problems people have when making bath bombs and how to either prevent or resolve these issues.

The Bombs Flatten and Soften
If this is the case, then you have too much water in the mixture and need to add some more of the dry ingredients in the correct ratio. Alternatively, you can add some white clay to your bath bombs which will have the same effect.

The Bombs Crumble or Dent
This is usually down to the fact you are not firming your mixture down into the mold enough, so all you need to do is push the mixture down harder, so it is denser. Sometimes, the additional ingredients can impact the consistency of the mixture. You may need to adjust the amount of water or extra ingredients until you get the right consistency that will retain its shape.

Bombs Crack as They Dry
This is because there is too much water in the mixture or sometimes it is from drying the bath bombs too fast. Add more dry mixture or use less water until you get the correct consistency. If they are drying too quickly, try leaving them somewhere cooler so they do not dry so fast.

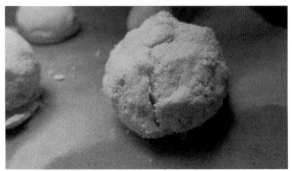

A cracked bath bomb

Bombs Fall Apart or Split on the Seam
This is often down to you not having the right amount of water in your mixture so add a little bit more and that should solve the problem. It can also be because you haven't held the molds together long enough or packed them full enough so that the two halves can join together. There needs to be a little bit more mixture than required in each half of the mold so that the two parts can attach firmly.

It Won't Come Out of the Mold
This will be because there is too much water or too much corn starch in the mixture. The latter is sticky and will cling to the mold, particularly if the molds are older. If done properly, the bombs should fall out of the mold and not require prising out.

The Mixture Comes Out of The Sides of the Mold
This means that you have added too much water to the mixture. Put the mixture back into the bowl, add more citric acid and bicarbonate of soda in the right proportions, and stir well. If you have added too much liquid, you will be able to see the mixture expanding in the bowl. This can be recovered because it will stop expanding. When it does, either put it in the molds or shape the bombs by hand and leave to dry. Sure, they won't be sellable, but you can still use them in your bath where they will have a lovely effect.

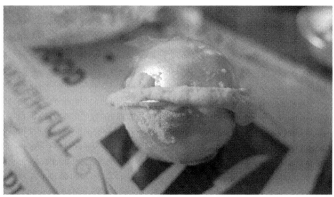

A bath bomb continuing to foam when put into the mold

Molding Tips

Molding is where most people have problems with their bath bombs and usually, if you are having problems with the molds, it is down to the consistency of the mixture. However, because this part of the process can be tricky here are some tips which should help solve some of the more commonly encountered problems.

Use a Round or Smooth Mold

If you use a mold that has sharp corners or edges, then you are going to find it hard to get the bath bomb out in one piece. Bath bomb molds with smoother edges are much easier for you to get the bombs out of. For example, if you are using an ice cube tray then get one that has rounded corners as the finished bath bombs will come out much easier. Square, star and other shapes with hard edges are going to be difficult to get the bath bomb out from.

Keep Them Small

The larger the bath bomb, the harder it is for it to stay together, so when you are starting out it is much better to make smaller bath bombs as they are easier to handle and succeed with. Smaller bath bombs dry faster and more consistently than larger ones and so are more likely to remain together.

Be Firm but Gentle

Pushing your mixture into a mold should be relatively easy and you don't need any superhuman strength to make them compact properly. If you feel that it is too much effort pushing your bath bombs into molds then there is a problem with your mixture. Check the consistency and add more water or dry mixture as required.

Drying Your Bath Bombs

Once you take the bath bombs out of the molds you want to leave them somewhere to dry for 24 to 48 hours. During this time leave them alone; don't prod, poke, or even move them. Just leave them be and they will dry and then you can move them and store them. Larger bath bombs will require more drying time than smaller ones.

Wrapping Your Bath Bombs

Once they have dried fully then you can wrap your bath bombs and store them somewhere clean and dry to preserve them and stop them from absorbing moisture and crumbling. Wrap and seal them in plastic wrap or bags so that they do not absorb moisture from the atmosphere which could then cause them to disintegrate.

ADDITIONAL INGREDIENTS FOR HEAVENLY BATH BOMBS

We talked about some of the additional ingredients you can use for your bath bombs earlier, but now we are going to go into more detail about the wide variety of ingredients that you can use to make your bath bombs more interesting. Some of these ingredients will benefit your skin whereas others just make the bath bomb look better and the bath itself more interesting.

Rather than add lots of ingredients to one bath bomb you should create different bath bombs with different sets of ingredients. Adding too many ingredients to a single bath bomb can make it very difficult for you to get the right consistency so it sets properly.

Sodium Lauryl Sulfoacetate

This is a powder which, when added to your bath bombs, make them foam so you get more of a bubble bath experience. It helps to soften the water and is very gentle. At a concentration of 3% it will not irritate your eyes and even up to 70% it will not irritate your skin. Typically, you will add up 10% concentration in a bath bomb.

Dead Sea Salts

These are mineral rich salts which are found in a lot of beauty products and are very therapeutic for your skin. You can use up to a 25% in your dry ingredients, though make sure you get the consistency right as they can absorb water.

Carrier Oils

These are high in vitamins and are fabulous at nourishing your skin, no matter what type of skin you have. Typically, used up to 5% concentration with your ingredients, though adjust the amount of water you use as too much liquid will mean your bath bombs don't hold together. Remember that because these are oil, they will float on top of the bath water rather than mix with it. Any essential oils that you use will also stick to the oil and therefore the skin. Be careful when using oils as they can make your bath slippery, so you need to take extra care getting in and out.

Epsom Salts

Adding these to your bath bombs makes for a great therapeutic soak for sore muscles; ideal for anyone who engages in sports! Use up to 25% in your dry ingredients mix, remembering to adjust water quantities to take into account the salts in the mixture.

Essential Oils

These are used to add the smell to your bath bombs and are natural products, extracted from plants and herbs. The different essential oils have a wide variety of therapeutic properties and you need to consider the properties of the oils when adding other ingredients to your bath bombs. There is no point adding an oil which promotes relaxation to a bath bomb that contains something which is invigorating.

Essential oils are concentrated so you do not need a large amount in your bath bombs, typically six to eight drops will be plenty. Just remember that adding these oils will reduce the amount of water you need to achieve the right consistency.

Here's some of the most popular oils and their properties. There are many other oils out there as well as fragrance oils, which are weaker than essential oils but often are blended or artificial aromas. Be aware that some people can suffer with skin irritation from both fragrance and essential oils, so ensure bath bombs are labelled if selling or you perform a skin test if using them yourself.

- Lavender – this is a very popular fragrance which is renowned for its relaxing effects. It is good for almost all skin types though a few people do find it irritates their skin – try a little on your skin first if you are unsure. It blends very well with most oils, though is particularly good with citrus, woody, and pine oils, as well as rose, rosemary and ylang ylang.
- Rosemary – a very invigorating oil, suitable for most skin types, though it is particularly good for oily skin. It blends well with most oils, including pine, herbals and wood oils.

- Peppermint – another refreshing fragrance which is stimulating, yet cooling, helping to clear the sinuses. It is good for most skin types and blends well with the majority of oils.
- Lemon – a very popular fragrance with an uplifting effect that is great for oily skin or people suffering from acne. This is best used at a low concentration as it is quite strong and blends well with a gentler oil, such as lavender or chamomile.
- Grapefruit – an uplifting oil which is particularly good for oily or congested skin. It is one of the gentler members of the citrus family, though should still be used in low concentrations and combined with a gentler oil.
- Ylang Ylang – an exotic oil with a definite floral fragrance which has a very calming yet aphrodisiac effect. It is suitable for all skin types and blends well with almost all oils, particularly floral, wood and citrus oils.
- Pettigrain – a floral fragrance from the citrus family that is known to be both calming and uplifting. Unlike other citrus oils, this comes from leaves and so is less irritating than other oils from the same family. It is particularly good for congested skin types.
- Vanilla – a deep, sweet fragrance that is known to be very calming, though you don't need much as it is a very concentrated. It is excellent for all skin types and blends particularly well with floral and citrus oils.
- Roman Chamomile – a very deep, clean fragrance which has both a calming and a sedative effective. It is a very gentle oil and is good for children and sensitive skin types.

This are just some of the most common essential oils, though there are plenty more out there you can experiment with if you want. Just remember that many essential oils can increase your blood pressure, so if you are suffering with high blood pressure you need to be especially careful when choosing an oil.

Petals

These don't particularly have a therapeutic value, but they look fantastic and can really add to the perceived luxury of the resulting bath. The petals can add some scent, to the bath too with the most commonly used petals being rose, lavender, heather, jasmine and calendula. These can be bought online or found at some of the larger craft stores. Add up to 10% petals to your dry mixture, adjusting water used appropriately.

Herbs

These are great to add to your bath bombs and can be bought online or from some health food stores or craft stores. The most commonly used herbs include lemongrass, chamomile, eucalyptus, neem and green tea, all of which should be used in a concentration of no more than 10%. Adding these to your bath bomb brings a touch of herbal healing to your bath.

Seeds & Grains

These are great for exfoliating your skin as they both cleanse and get rid of any dry skin. The seeds can make for some great decoration, particularly if the bath bomb is rolled in them. Again, use a concentration of no more than 10%. Popular seeds to use include ground olive stones, ground almond stones, orange peel, lemon peel, sesame seeds or blue poppy seeds.

There are plenty more ingredients that you can add to your bath bomb, you are literally only limited by your imagination. Just make sure that anything you use is safe for humans and not toxic in any way. If you are selling your bath bombs, then ensure that they are clearly labelled with all the ingredients in case a buyer has an allergy or suffers with skin irritation.

Be careful on the concentration levels as too much of these ingredients can prevent the bath bomb from fizzing properly. Remember that the amount of water required to get the correct consistency will vary depending on the additional ingredients you use. Getting it right can involve some trial and error until you are used to using these extra ingredients and then you will find it easier.

These extra ingredients can make your bath bombs much more interesting, but can also be used to help mental, physical or emotional complaints. Lavender added to bath bombs, for example, can help someone who is stressed relax. Other ingredients can help smooth skin inflammation and provide much needed relief to a sufferer. Adding these extra ingredients can help you and it can make your bath bombs much more attractive to potential buyers too. It allows you to tailor make bath bombs based on someone's individual requirements.

BATH BOMB RECIPES

This chapter is devoted to a wide variety of bath bombs with all the recipes you have been waiting for. You know the basic recipe and probably have lots of ideas for adjusting these recipes to make them your own. Enjoy making these bath bombs and enjoy experimenting with the recipes!

Feel free to adjust the recipes, change the colorings or oils to make them right for your specific requirements. At the end of the day, you are the one using the bath bombs and you want them to be ideal for you. I would recommend tracking your changes to the recipes in a notebook so that you know what you have added to the mixture. This means that when you make the perfect bath bomb, you know exactly what you did and can replicate the process. It also means that when things go wrong, you know exactly what it is that went wrong.

There are plenty of different recipes here, so there is something for everyone. You may find it easier to start with the simpler recipes and then move on to the more advanced ones once you are used to getting the right consistency.

Easter Egg Bath Bombs

These are great bath bombs for Easter, but the shape is easy to make and are popular all year round. You can shape these using egg shaped plastic contains such as those you buy some brands of women's tights in, Kinder Eggs or children's toys.

Ingredients:
- 1 cup baking soda
- ½ cup Epsom salts
- ½ cup corn starch powder
- ½ cup citric acid
- 8-10 tablespoons carrier oil
- 2 teaspoons of peppermint and lavender oil
- 6 to 9 drops of food coloring

Method:
1. Mix the dry ingredients together and then separate equally into three bowls
2. To each bowl add two tablespoons of carrier oil plus two or three drops of food coloring, mixing well and quickly (the food coloring and citric acid will react together which is why you need to be fast)
3. The mixture should be crumbly but not soaking wet, i.e. you can squeeze it together so it clumps but it still crumbles when you rub it between your fingers
4. Scoop the mixture into the plastic eggs and pack it tightly. If you over fill each half, then the excess mixture will come out as you close the mold and can be brushed away and reused
5. Leave the bath bomb in the mold for five to ten minutes, then slide the top half of the mold off, squeezing the sides gently and using a screwing motion
6. Repeat with the bottom and you should have a great looking egg-shaped bath bomb
7. Leave the bath bombs for two days on a towel to dry
8. If the egg crumbles when you take it out, then put it back in the bowl and dry again and if the two halves don't stick together properly add some more oil

Bath Cookies

These are an interesting variation on the bath bomb and because they are small balls they are much easier to mold, being very forgiving of problems with the mixture consistency. These bath bombs can be decorated with things like cloves, dried orange or lemon peel and more to make them more interesting.

Ingredients:

- 2 cups sea salt (finely ground)
- ½ cup corn starch
- ½ cup baking soda
- 2 eggs
- 2 tablespoons of light oil
- 1 teaspoon vitamin E oil
- 5 or 6 drops essential oil (any you like)

Method:

1. Preheat your oven to 350F/175C
2. Mix together all the ingredients in a glass bowl
3. Scoop out a teaspoon of the mixture and roll it into a 1" ball then place on an ungreased cookie sheet
4. Repeat until all the dough is used up
5. Bake in your oven for 10 minutes until they are lightly browned
6. Leave the "cookies" to cool on a wire rack and then store in an airtight container

Cupcakes

Presenting your bath bombs as cupcakes is a fantastic idea and they look amazing, though it does require a little bit more work on your part! Here is an ideal opportunity for you to allow your imagination to run riot as you decorate and color your "cupcakes" with bath friendly items to them look stunning. Instead of making the actual cupcake just one color you can layer the colors to make them look better plus you can decorate the "frosting" with a variety of herbs, petals and other decorations.

Ingredients:

- 2 cups baking soda
- 1 cup citric acid
- 1 tablespoon almond oil (you can use other oils such as grapeseed or olive)
- 1 teaspoon Bentonite clay (makes the bath bombs firmer)
- 5 drops essential oil of your choice
- 3 to 5 drops food coloring
- 1 teaspoon Sodium Lauryl Sulfate (can use up to a tablespoon if you want more lather from your bath bombs)
- Witch hazel (in a spray bottle)
- Paper cupcake liners
- Silicone cupcake molds

Method:

1. Place the paper liners inside the mold in preparation (a deep cupcake baking tray will do just fine)
2. Mix all the dry ingredients together carefully in a large glass bowl, though try not to breathe in too much of the dry ingredients as it can irritate some people in this form (it is perfectly safe in the bath)
3. Add your essential oils and coloring to the dry mixture and stir well but gently
4. Knead the mixture with one hand, as if you were making bread, and spray it with witch hazel, being careful not to get the dough too wet
5. Continue to knead and spray until it has the consistency of a crumbly dough
6. Divide the mixture between the paper cupcake lines and pack the mixture down firmly
7. Leave to set for ten minutes before removing

Cupcake Bath Bomb Frosting

This is the recipe for a frosting you can use on these bath bombs, though you can swirl the colors and be imaginative here!

Ingredients:

- 1lb/454g powdered sugar
- 5 or 6 tablespoons warm water
- 3 tablespoons meringue powder or powdered egg whites
- ¼ teaspoon cream of tartar
- Some food coloring
- Some essential oils (optional but make sure they complement the oils in the cupcake itself)

Method:

1. Mix the meringue powder and warm water together in a glass bowl
2. Add the sugar and cream of tartar
3. Beat using a hand mixer on a high speed, though if it feels like a stiff cookie dough add an additional tablespoon of water
4. Beat for between seven and nine minutes until it forms stiff peaks and looks thick and fluffy
5. Add the essential oils and coloring and beat for another minute until well mixed
6. Decorate your cupcakes with the frosting using a cake frosting bag
7. Leave overnight to harden before packaging or storing and be sure your family know not to eat them!

Fizzy Lemon Bath Bombs

Lemons are well known to be detoxifying and to have astringent qualities which are very rejuvenating to the skin, can help reduce blemishes and makes your skin look less tired. This recipe makes bath bombs that are perfect for de-stressing after a hard day!

Ingredients:
- 1 cup baking soda
- ½ cup citric acid
- 10 drops lemon essential oil
- Zest from 1 lemon (unwaxed is best)
- Witch hazel in a spray bottle

Method:
1. Dry the lemon zest out in your oven for a few minutes at 350F/175C – it is ready when it darkens, becomes more intense in color and starts to curl up. This ensures the moisture in the zest doesn't interfere in the bath bomb drying process
2. In a glass bowl, mix together the citric acid and baking soda until well combined
3. Add half the zest and the lemon oil
4. Spray everything lightly with the witch hazel and continue to mix until it reaches the right consistency
5. Press the mixture into your molds as soon as the consistency is correct using a firm pressure and leave to dry at room temperature until solid then remove and continue to dry on paper towels
6. You can decorate the drying bath bombs with some more of the lemon zest if you would like

Relaxing Bath Bomb

This is a wonderful bath bomb to relax with and let the stress of the day drain away, also being very rejuvenating for your skin.

Ingredients:

- 8oz/226g baking soda
- 4oz/113g Epsom salts
- 4oz/113g corn starch
- 4oz/113g cream of tartar
- 2 teaspoons coconut oil
- 2 teaspoons lavender oil
- ¾ teaspoon water
- Purple food coloring

Method:

1. Mix all the dry ingredients in a large glass bowl
2. In a separate small glass bowl mix together the oil, food coloring and water
3. Combine the wet and dry ingredients and mix well until the color is evenly distributed throughout the mixture and it reaches the right consistency (add more water a few drops at a time if necessary)
4. Pack the mixture into your molds firmly
5. Leave to dry for 24 hours, though depending on the shape of your mold you can remove them earlier and leave them to dry on a towel

Foamy Madness

These bath bombs are pretty awesome to use and foam like crazy in your bath, but they do take some time to make, about a week including all the waiting but it is worth it. Don't be tempted to try and speed the process up as you can ruin your bath bombs if you do.

Ingredients:
- 4 cups baking soda
- ½ cup thick, unscented shampoo or body wash
- ½ cup citric acid
- 4 tablespoons olive oil

Method:
1. Mix the baking soda and shampoo together in a glass bowl until well combined
2. Put the mixture into a large shallow container such as a cookie sheet with an edge and leave for 2 or 3 days for the water to evaporate. If it isn't dry, then leave it another 24 hours as the water in the shampoo will react with the citric acid
3. Pour this mixture back into a bowl and add the citric acid, mixing well
4. Add the oil and mix until well combined, often you have to use your hands here
5. Squeeze the mixture into shapes with your hands and then leave on wax paper for 2 or 3 days to dry fully – do not disturb them during the drying time
6. Store your bath bombs in an air tight, dry container

Green Tea Delight

Green tea is well known to be high in anti-oxidants which are very beneficial to your skin. This recipe uses Epsom salts as well, which have a whole host of other benefits for your skin. For this recipe you want a powdered green tea which you can find online or from Asian markets. You won't need a large amount, but any leftover will make for a rejuvenating drink! This is a great bath bomb for rejuvenating your skin and helping you feel great.

Ingredients:
- 1 cup baking soda
- ½ cup citric acid
- ½ cup corn starch
- ½ cup Epsom salts
- 2 tablespoons almond oil
- 2 tablespoons powdered green tea
- 2 teaspoons water
- ½ teaspoon essential oil (optional)

Method:
1. In a glass bowl, mix together the green tea powder, citric acid, corn starch, and Epsom salts
2. Add the rest of the ingredients and mix thoroughly
3. Line a muffin tin with paper liners
4. Fill each liner with bath bomb mixture and press down, topping up with more mixture and pressing down again, smoothing the tops
5. Leave to dry for 4 or 5 hours
6. Once they are firm you can blow or shake off any crumbs from the top of the bath bomb before using or storing

Magic Confetti Bath Bombs

These are fantastic bath bombs and you can use different types of confetti depending on colors you are using or any special occasions, e.g. Valentine's Day, or even add petals or herbs to the mixture.

Ingredients:
- 2 parts sodium bicarbonate
- 1 part citric acid
- Handful of confetti
- Small amount of water or witch hazel
- Coloring / essential oils as required

Method:
1. Mix the dry ingredients together in a glass bowl until well combined
2. Spray with water and mix, continuing to spray until the right consistency has been achieved
3. Pack the mixture firmly into your molds and leave to dry for 30 to 60 minutes until you can remove them from the molds
4. Leave the bath bombs on a towel to dry overnight before storing

Rose Petal Love

Nothing says, "I love you" like roses and rose petals added to a bath bomb make for a luxurious and relaxing bath. The addition of rose petals makes these ideal for Valentine's Day or as a gift to a loved one. This recipe should make enough for around seven medium sized bath bombs.

Ingredients:
- 1½ cups baking soda
- ½ cup citric acid
- ¼ cup dried rose petals
- ½ tablespoon water
- 2 teaspoons almond oil
- 10 to 15 drops rose oil (can be a fragrant oil rather than essential)
- 5 drops of red or pink food coloring

Method:
1. Mix all the dry ingredients together in a glass bowl until well combined
2. Add the almond oil, coloring, and rose oil, stirring until thoroughly mixed
3. Add the water and stir again – if the mixture is not at the right consistency then add more water, a little at a time, until it is
4. Pack the mixture down into your molds and leave for an hour or two (depending on the mold size) until they can be removed
5. Leave on wax paper for another day or two until completely dry before storing

Relaxing Rose and Chamomile Bath Bomb

This is a great variation on the above bath bomb that adds chamomile to the mix which is really relaxing and de-stressing.

Ingredients:

- 1½ cups bicarbonate of soda
- ½ cup citric acid
- 2 tablespoons almond oil
- Handful of dried chamomile flowers
- Handful of dried rose petals
- 14 drops rose essential oil
- 4 drops lavender essential oil

Method:

1. Mix the dry ingredients together in a glass bowl
2. In a separate bowl, mix together the rose and lavender oils with the almond oil and any food coloring you are using
3. Mix the wet and dry ingredients together and check the consistency – you may need to add more water or oil depending on the quantities of dried flowers used
4. Press the mixture down firmly into your molds and leave to dry for 48 hours before gently removing and storing

Lavender and Oatmeal Bath Bomb

This is a great recipe for some very relaxing bath bombs; the recipe should produce three good sized bath bombs. The oatmeal is very good for your skin and the lavender provides some much needed relaxation.

Ingredients:
- 1 cup baking soda
- ½ cup citric acid
- ¼ cup quick oats
- ¼ teaspoon lavender essential oil
- ⅛ teaspoon rose geranium essential oil
- Handful each of lavender flowers and rose petals
- Witch hazel in a spray bottle

Method:
1. Mix the baking soda and citric acid together in a bowl
2. Add the oats and stir well until thoroughly combined
3. Add the essential oils and mix well, ensuring the oils are evenly distributed
4. Spray with witch hazel until it reaches the right consistency – spray a little at a time to ensure you don't add too much
5. Press the mixture firmly into your bath bomb molds (you can sprinkle some dried flowers on the inside of the molds first so that they cover the outside of the bombs)
6. Try to hollow out a part of the bath bomb and put some dried flowers in to this hole, covering it with more of the mixture
7. Leave to dry for a few hours (depending on the size of the mold) and then remove, leaving for a further 24 hours to dry on wax paper

Therapeutic Coconut Oil Bath Bombs

Coconut oil is very good for your skin and this recipe combines the benefits of this oil with the relaxation associated with Epsom salts to make a wonderfully therapeutic bath bomb.

Ingredients:
- 1 cup baking soda
- ½ cup arrowroot powder
- ½ cup citric acid
- 2 tablespoons coconut oil
- 2 tablespoons Epsom salts
- 5 teaspoons water
- 10 to 15 drops essential oil of your choice
- Food coloring

Method:
1. Mix the dry ingredients together in a large glass bowl
2. Whisk in the coconut oil until you end up with a sand like mixture
3. Add the water, coloring and essential oils (start with less water so you don't overdo it) and stir well until thoroughly combined
4. Push the mixture firmly down in to your molds and leave to dry for a few hours (depending on the size of the molds) before turning out on to wax paper and leaving to dry for a further 24 hours before storing

Aromatherapy Shower Bomb

This is a variation on the bath bomb that is used while in the shower. The shower bomb is placed in the corner of your shower out of the water and slowly breaks down in the steam, releasing the aromatherapy oils from it. You can use any oils you want, though eucalyptus and menthol are particularly good for clearing your sinuses.

Ingredients:
- 1 cup baking soda
- ¼ cup (sometimes less) water
- 3 to 4 drops of essential oils (2 drops each of eucalyptus, peppermint and lavender makes for a great cold busting bomb)

Method:
1. Put the baking soda in a large glass bowl and slowly add the water until it becomes a thick paste
2. Add the essential oils and mix until they are evenly distributed
3. Squeeze the paste into ball shapes (remember not to add too much water but if you do, add some more baking soda) and it should hold its shape, feeling dry to the touch
4. Press the mixture firmly down into the molds and leave to dry before removing and leaving for another 24 hours to dry on wax paper

Ocean Fresh Bath Bomb

This is a lovely refreshing bath bomb that is positively rejuvenating for your skin. Full of vitamins and minerals together with a divine smell you are going to love bringing the spirit of the ocean into your bathroom!

Ingredients:
- 1 cup baking soda
- ½ cup citric acid
- ¼ cup sea salt
- 2 to 4 ounces of 86% witch hazel
- 2 tablespoons kelp powder
- 2 tablespoons coral calcium powder
- ⅛ teaspoon each of mandarin, spearmint, juniper and grapefruit oils

Method:
1. Thoroughly combine the sea salt, kelp powder, baking soda, and coral calcium in a large glass bowl
2. Add the essential oils and stir until they are evenly distributed, breaking up any clumps
3. Add the citric acid and stir well
4. Spray with the witch hazel as you mix until it reaches the right consistency
5. Mold into shape or press firmly into your molds, leaving for around four hours before removing, then dry overnight on wax paper

Avocado Bath Bomb

Avocado is full of vitamins that are essential for healthy skin. Easy to make, this recipe will produce four large bath bombs or can be molded into shapes to produce more smaller ones.

Ingredients:

- 1lb/454g baking soda
- ½lb/227g citric acid
- ½oz/14g fresh, ripe avocado (remove any peel)
- ½oz/14g olive oil
- ½ teaspoon green mineral oxide
- 30 drops rosewood essential oil
- 25 drops bergamot essential oil
- 25 drops lemongrass essential oil

Method:

1. In a large glass bowl, mix together the green oxide, citric acid and baking soda
2. In a separate bowl, mix together the avocado and olive oil; you may want to use a blender or hand mixer to ensure the mixture is smooth
3. Combine the two mixtures and stir thoroughly
4. Add the essential oils and some extra water, if necessary, to get the right consistency and stir well
5. Fill the molds, pressing down firmly and leave to dry for a few hours before removing and leaving to dry overnight on wax paper

Sinus Clearing Bath Bomb

This great mixture releases a lovely aroma which is superb for clearing your sinuses and is very refreshing. Definitely one to try and one you will enjoy, particularly if you are feeling under the weather or suffering with a cold.

Ingredients:

- ¾ cup corn starch
- ½ cup citric acid
- ¼ cup granulated sugar
- A dash of baking soda
- 1 teaspoon eucalyptus essential oil
- 1 teaspoon tangerine essential oil
- ½ teaspoon frankincense essential oil

Method:

1. Mix the baking soda, citric acid, sugar, and corn starch in a glass mixing bowl
2. Add the essential oils and whisk to ensure it is thoroughly blended
3. Spray with water until you reach the right consistency
4. Press firmly into your mold and leave to dry for a few hours before turning it out on to wax paper to dry overnight

Fizzy Chocolate Cupcakes

Decidedly decadent bath bombs that are luxurious and relaxing, though you may come out of the bath wanting a candy bar!

Ingredients:
- ½ cup Epsom salts
- ½ cup baking soda
- ¼ cup raw cacao powder
- ¼ cup citric acid
- ½ teaspoon almond oil (you can substitute with coconut or olive oil if you prefer)
- ½ teaspoon vanilla essence

Method:
1. In a large glass bowl, mix together the dry ingredients
2. In a separate bowl, blend the vanilla essence and the oil
3. Combine the wet and dry mixtures, stirring well until thoroughly combined
4. Either add to the bath as a powder or shape into a bath bomb following the usual procedure

Perfect Pear Bombs

These are an unusual bath bomb as pear aromas are not common. However, the aroma is very pleasant, and it works well to relax you in the bath. It is well worth a try because it is very different to normal bath bombs. These are particularly good as bath bombs to sell if you can find molds in the shape of the pear fruit.

Ingredients:

- 1 cup baking soda
- 1 cup corn starch
- 1 cup citric acid
- ¼ cup Epsom salts
- Green food coloring
- Pear fragrance or essential oil

Method:

1. Combine the dry ingredients in a large glass bowl until thoroughly mixed
2. Add several drops of the pear fragrance, stirring well until it has a strong enough scent for you
3. Add a few drops of food coloring to get the right shade of green
4. Spray carefully with water and stir until you get the right consistency
5. Press firmly into your mold (or shape by hand) and leave for a few hours before removing from the mold and leaving to dry overnight on wax paper

Perfect Peppermint

This is a great, refreshing bath bomb that will leave you feeling invigorating while clearing out your sinuses. Perfect for when you have a cold, allergies, or just need a bit of a kick.

Ingredients:
- 1 cup baking soda
- ½ cup citric acid
- 2 tablespoons jojoba oil (you can substitute with almond, olive or coconut oil)
- 1 tablespoon witch hazel
- 5 drops each of peppermint, eucalyptus and lemon essential oil

Method:
1. In a large glass bowl, mix together the baking soda and citric acid
2. Add both the oil and essential oils, then mix well
3. Add in the witch hazel, stirring constantly to prevent the ingredients fizzing up – adding a little at a time until you get the right consistency
4. Press the mixture firmly into your molds, leaving for a few hours before turning out on to wax paper and leaving to dry overnight

Relaxing Lavender

This is probably my favorite bath bomb, being so relaxing. It is great to use after a long, stressful day and can be dyed purple using coloring if you would like, though adjust the water quantity appropriately. Lavender is a very popular scent and one that most people like, it's great for gifts of sales.

Ingredients:
- 1 cup baking soda
- ½ cup corn starch
- ½ cup citric acid
- 4 tablespoons dried lavender flowers
- 3 tablespoons Epsom salts
- 2 teaspoons almond oil
- ¾ teaspoon water
- 15 drops lavender essential oil

Method:
1. In a large glass bowl, mix together the dry ingredients until well combined
2. In a separate smaller bowl, mix the essential oil and almond oil with a little of the water and any food coloring
3. Pour the wet mixture into the dry and stir well until combined
4. Add more water, a little at a time until you reach the right consistency
5. Press firmly into your molds, leaving for a few hours before removing and turning out on to wax paper to dry overnight

Winter Warmer

The winter months are toughest on your skin, with the cold, harsh weather and the rain or snow taking its toll. Keeping your skin well-nourished is a particular challenge in these colder months, but this bath bomb is going to help soothe your stress and moisturize your skin. You can add some Epsom salts or even Dead Sea salts to make the bath bomb extra relaxing and nourishing.

Ingredients:

- 1 cup baking soda
- ½ cup citric acid
- 2½ tablespoons coconut oil or melted shea butter
- ½ tablespoon of either jojoba, almond, avocado or grapeseed oil
- ½ teaspoon vitamin E oil
- 15-20 drops of essential oil – choose your favorite relaxing or soothing oil
- A few drops of food coloring of your choice

Method:

1. In a large glass bowl, mix together the citric acid and baking soda
2. In a separate bowl, mix together all the wet ingredients, stirring well
3. Combine the wet and dry ingredients, mixing until well combined
4. Spray with witch hazel until you get the right consistency
5. Press firmly into your molds and leave to dry for a few hours before turning out on to wax paper, leaving them overnight to finish drying

Sea Salt Refresh

Sea salt is very rejuvenating for your skin, helping to remove dead skin amongst other things. This bath bomb is super relaxing and has a wonderful effect on your skin; well worth a try!

Ingredients:
- 1 cup baking soda
- ½ cup citric acid
- ¼ cup fine non-iodized sea salt
- 10 – 15 drops of Orange essential oil
- Course pink salt to garnish

Method:
1. Put the pink salt into your mold first as it will be the decoration on the outside of your bath bombs
2. In a large glass bowl, mix together the sea salt, baking soda, and citric acid until well combined
3. Add the essential oil and mix well
4. Spray with witch hazel, stirring constantly, until the right consistency is reached
5. Press firmly into your molds, leaving a few hours before turning out on to wax paper to dry overnight

Sage and Lemongrass

This is an unusual bath bomb that is both pleasant and relaxing. With a deep green color, it is particularly attractive and looks great as a gift! Due to the color these work very well in leaf shaped molds and can be shaped for festive seasons, e.g. as Christmas trees.

Ingredients:
- 4½oz/128g baking soda
- 2¼oz/64g citric acid
- 1oz/28g Argan oil
- ½oz/14g kaolin or white cosmetic clay
- ½ teaspoon lemongrass and sage fragrance oil
- Chromium green oxide powder (for coloring)

Method:
1. In a large glass bowl, mix together the dry ingredients
2. Add the wet ingredients to the mixture and stir until thoroughly combined
3. Spray with witch hazel, a little at a time, until the right consistency is reached
4. Press firmly into your mold and leave for a few hours before turning out on to wax paper and drying overnight

Geranium and Rose

These two scents make for a wonderful combination that is absolutely divine. Feel free to adjust the recipe to use other oils or salts depending on your skin type or requirements.

Ingredients:

- 1 cup baking soda
- ½ cup Epsom salts
- ½ cup citric acid
- 1 tablespoon rose water
- 1 teaspoon olive oil
- 20 drops geranium essential oil
- Handful dried rose petals

Method:

1. In a large glass bowl, mix the dry ingredients together
2. Add the olive oil and essential oil whilst stirring constantly
3. Add the rose petals and stir until they are evenly dispersed
4. Spray with witch hazel or water until you reach the right consistency, it may need a little more than normal due to the petals in the mixture
5. Pack firmly into your molds and leave to dry for a few hours before turning them out on to wax paper and leave them to dry for up to a week (the rose petals will absorb moisture and need to dry thoroughly)

Ginger Snaps

These are wonderfully scented bath bombs that are almost good enough to eat! You can shape these into gingerbread men or cookie shapes or use more traditional bath bomb molds.

Ingredients:
- 2 cups baking soda
- 1 cup citric acid
- ½oz/14g gingersnap cookie fragrance oil
- 40 drops brown soap coloring

Method:
1. In a large glass bowl, mix together the baking soda and citric acid until thoroughly combined
2. Add the oil and coloring, then stir well
3. Spray with witch hazel, a little at a time, until the mixture reaches the right consistency
4. Shape by hand or press firmly into your molds
5. Leave in the mold for a few hours before turning out on to wax paper
6. If shaped by hand leave on wax paper overnight to dry thoroughly

Ginger Peach Delight

An unusual combination of fragrances that makes for a delightful bath bomb that is very enjoyable.

Ingredients:

- 8oz/227g baking soda
- 4oz/128g citric acid
- 4oz/128g corn starch
- 4oz/128g Dead Sea salt
- 2½ tablespoons cherry kernel oil
- ¾ tablespoon water
- 2 teaspoons ginger peach fragrance oil
- 2 drops yellow food coloring
- 1 drop red food coloring

Method:

1. Mix all the dry ingredients together in a large glass bowl until smooth
2. In a separate bowl, whisk the wet ingredients together
3. Add the wet ingredients to the dry, stirring constantly, breaking up any lumps that form (adding the liquid too quickly or not stirring enough will cause the mixture to foam)
4. Check the consistency and add more water (a little at a time) until it is correct
5. Press down firmly into your molds and leave for a few hours to dry before turning out on to wax paper and leaving to dry overnight

Coconut Oil and White Tea

This is an interesting combination that works surprisingly well. You can color these however you want or even divide the mixture into two or three parts, coloring each part separately before layering the different colors in your mold.

Ingredients:

- 1 cup baking soda
- ½ cup corn starch
- ½ cup citric acid
- 2 tablespoons coconut oil
- 2 tablespoons Epsom salts
- 4 or 5 teaspoons brewed and cooled white tea (make it very strong)
- A few drops of essential oils of your choice
- A few drops of food coloring of your choice

Method:

1. In a large glass bowl, mix together the citric acid, salts, corn starch and baking soda
2. Whisk in the coconut oil until it takes on a sandy texture
3. Add the coloring and essential oils, stirring until evenly dispersed
4. Add the white tea to the mixture a teaspoon at a time, stirring as you do until it reaches the right consistency
5. Pack firmly into your mold, leaving a few hours before removing and turning out on to wax paper to dry overnight

Tangerine Dream
A very uplifting bath bomb which is also great for your skin!

Ingredients:
- 2 cups baking soda
- 1 cup Epsom salt
- 1 cup citric acid
- 2 tablespoons cocoa butter (meted)
- 2 tablespoons sweet almond oil
- 5 to 8 drops of tangerine essential oil
- Small handful of orange or tangerine zest (dried in your oven)

Method:
1. Mix the dry ingredients together in a glass bowl until thoroughly combined
2. In a separate bowl, mix together the melted cocoa butter, the oil and the essential oils plus any food coloring
3. Add the water, a little at a time until you get the right consistency
4. Shape by hand or press firmly into molds, leaving for a few hours before turning out on to wax paper to dry overnight

Cleansing Apricot Bath Bombs

This is a very cleansing recipe that is good for your skin. Feel free to add some ground apricot kernels to the mixture or even use apricot kernel oil instead of some of the water.

Ingredients:
- 1 cup baking soda
- 1 cup citric acid
- 1 cup corn starch
- ¼ cup Epsom salts
- Apricot fragrance oil
- Orange food coloring

Method:
1. Mix together the dry ingredients in a glass bowl until thoroughly combined
2. Add the fragrance oil and food coloring until the desired color and scent is achieved
3. Spray the mixture with water, stirring often until it is at the right consistency
4. Press firmly into your mold, leave for several hours before turning out on to wax paper to dry overnight

Tropical Bath Bomb

This is a bath bomb that is just packed full of goodness with vitamins A, C, E, B complexes and more as well as providing trace minerals for your skin. It is anti-aging, soothing to skin ailments, and very moisturizing, making it ideal for anyone who suffers from any skin complaints including eczema and psoriasis.

Ingredients:

- 1 cup baking soda
- ½ cup Epsom salts
- ½ cup citric acid
- ½ cup coconut milk powder
- 1 to 4 tablespoons mango powder
- 1 tablespoon almond oil
- 1 teaspoon aloe vera 200x powder
- 15 drops lime essential oil

Method:

1. In your food processor blend together the aloe powder, coconut milk powder, mango powder, baking soda, and citric acid with the essential oil before transferring to a large glass bowl
2. In your food processor, blend together the almond oil and Epsom salts, then add to the baking soda mixture, stirring well
3. Spray with witch hazel (the mixture reacts less to this than water) until it reaches the right consistency
4. Pack firmly into your molds, leave for a few hours, then carefully remove and leave dry overnight on wax paper

Snowballs

These are an interesting bath bomb that will take three or four days to complete due to the drying time, but they make a fantastic gift in an ornate glass jar or wrapped. This recipe will make enough for around two large or four small balls. Dye the balls any color you want to fit in with your bathroom color scheme or gift scheme.

Ingredients:

- 2 cups Epson salts
- 2 tablespoons water
- 5 or 6 drops essential oil of your choice
- 1 to 3 drops food coloring

Method:

1. Mix together the Epsom salts and the water in a mixing bowl
2. Add the essential oil and food coloring until you get the desired scent and color, stirring well to ensure it is evenly dispersed
3. Press some mixture into half of a bath bomb mold, packing firmly then fill the second half
4. Press the two halves together then either tape or otherwise secure the halves together for half an hour
5. Remove the top part of the mold carefully then leave the bath bomb to stand overnight in the bottom half of the mold
6. Carefully remove the mold and leave to stand for a further two or three days until completely dry throughout then store

Tiger Bombs

These are very interesting looking bath bombs that make great gifts or can be kept and enjoyed yourself!

Ingredients:
- 4 cups baking soda
- 2 cups citric acid
- 1oz/28g buttercream fragrance oil
- 4 tablespoon kaolin clay
- 2 tablespoon cocoa butter
- 1 tablespoon cappuccino mica

Method:
1. In a large glass bowl, mix together the baking soda, clay, and citric acid, ensuring it is thoroughly mixed and any clumps are broken up (note you can sift the baking soda through a sieve to get rid of clumps)
2. Melt the cocoa butter and mix the fragrance oil into the liquid
3. Pour this into the dry ingredients and stir until thoroughly combined, breaking up any clumps
4. Divide the mixture evenly into two separate bowls
5. Add the cappuccino mica to one of the bowls and mix well
6. Check the consistency of both mixtures and spray with witch hazel until they are correct
7. Put a little of one color into one half of a spherical bath bomb mold, then some of the other color and repeat, pressing the layers down firmly
8. Repeat with the other half of the mold until both sides are full
9. Press the two halves together and use a gentle twisting motion (it does help if you overfill the molds then the mixture meets in the middle)
10. Leave the bomb for about an hour to solidify and then remove the top
11. Tip it over carefully and remove the other half of the mold
12. Leave on wax paper to dry for at least 24 hours before storing

Honey and Milk Delight

A truly pampering bath bomb that is absolutely heavenly and a great excuse to stay in the bath for ages! This recipe will produce enough mixture for around a dozen bath bombs. This technique of making bath bombs can be used with any complimentary combination to make a bath bomb of two different halves. If you are selling your bath bombs, then these can be very attractive and get a lot of attention, so can be worth the extra effort.

Ingredients:
- 2 cups baking soda
- 1 cup citric acid
- ½ cup powdered milk
- ½ cup corn starch
- 2 tablespoons extra-virgin olive oil (substitute for another carrier oil if you prefer)
- 2 tablespoons honey
- 4 teaspoons cocoa butter
- 2 teaspoons vanilla extract

Method:
1. In a large glass bowl, mix together the corn starch, powdered milk, citric acid and baking soda
2. Divide this mixture between two separate bowls
3. In a saucepan on a low heat melt two teaspoons of the cocoa butter together with a tablespoon of olive oil and the vanilla extract
4. Using your blender, blend one of the bowls of dry ingredients together with the ingredients from step 3 above. Put these to one side
5. In a clean saucepan, melt together the rest of the cocoa butter together with the honey and the rest of the olive oil
6. Blend this in your food processor with the other bowl of dry ingredients
7. Check the consistency of both mixtures is correct and if not then spray with witch hazel until they are
8. Pack one half of a bath bomb mold with the honey mixture and the other half with the milk mixture
9. Push both halves of the mold together, leaving a small gap in the middle of the bath bomb for the baking soda to rise
10. Leave for an hour to dry then remove from the mold (carefully) and place on wax paper for 24 hours to dry fully

Cocoa Butter Bomb

This is a really moisturizing bath bomb that is great for your skin, plus it has a good, long shelf life. This recipe will make enough for around five medium sized bath bombs.

Ingredients:
- 2 cups baking soda
- 1 cup citric acid
- 1 teaspoon melted cocoa butter
- 1 teaspoon essential oil of your choice

Method:
1. Mix all the ingredients together in a glass bowl until thoroughly combined
2. Spray with witch hazel until it reaches the right consistency
3. Shape by hand or pack firmly in molds (leave for a few hours in the mold before removing to ensure it has firmed enough)
4. Leave on wax paper for 24 hours to dry before storing

Spiced Rose Bomb

This is a very unusual bath bomb that combines a hint of exotic spices with that familiar, and favorite, scent of roses. It is colored naturally using beetroot powder, but you can substitute this for red food coloring if that is easier to get hold of.

Ingredients:

- 1 cup baking soda
- ½ cup Epsom salts
- ½ cup citric acid
- 1 tablespoon almond oil
- 1 teaspoon beetroot powder
- 10 drops lavender essential oil
- 5 drops cardamom essential oil
- 2 drops rose absolute

Method:

1. In a large glass bowl, mix together the baking soda, beetroot powder, and citric acid until well combined
2. In a separate bowl, mix together the essential oils, almond oil, and Epsom salts (using a food processor can help)
3. Combine the two sets of ingredients and stir well
4. Spray with witch hazel until it reaches the right consistency
5. Pack firmly into molds, leaving for a few hours before removing to dry on wax paper for 24 hours

Vanilla Rose

Another interesting combination of scents which makes for a heavenly bath bomb. The addition of oats helps smooth skin irritation and makes this ideal for anyone who suffers with dry skin.

Ingredients:
- 1 cup baking soda
- ½ cup citric acid
- ¼ cup Quaker porridge oats
- Pink food coloring
- Lavender, vanilla and rose essential oil
- Rose Water
- Handful of dried rose petals
- Handful of dried lavender leaves

Method:
1. Put the petals on the inside of your molds so they will stick to the outside of your bath bombs
2. In a large glass bowl, mix together the dry ingredients, ensuring there are no lumps
3. In a separate bowl, mix together the wet ingredients – use as much essential oil / coloring as you want
4. Combine the wet and dry ingredients, ensuring it is thoroughly mixed and there are no lumps
5. Spray with rose water (or witch hazel) until the right consistency is achieved
6. Push the mixture down firmly into the molds, leaving for a few hours to dry before turning out on to wax paper to dry overnight

Pink Salt Bath Melts

These bath bombs are wonderful in your bath, though they do not lather very well due to the high salt content. However, it is very luxurious, being both exfoliating and moisturizing. The Himalayan pink salt is very good for you and will help slough off any dead skin.

Ingredients:

- 32oz/908g shea butter (melted)
- 16oz/454g coarse Himalayan pink salt
- Essential oils of your choice
- Food coloring of your choice

Method:

1. Mix the coloring and essential oil into the melted Shea butter, stirring well
2. Add half the salt to the mixture and stir well, it will sink to the bottom of the bowl
3. Put some of the salt into each mold so it sticks to the outside and sinks into the bars
4. Pour the mixture into your molds and leave to cool for 3 to 4 hours before removing from them
5. Put the bar under running water or use it as soap to get the full benefit from the salt and shea butter

Fizzy Jasmine Bomb

This is a lovely bath bomb that uses the pleasant, yet unusual, scent of jasmine. It is very relaxing, and I do feel there is something special about this particular aroma. To make this extra special you can use some dried flowers in the molds, add some Epsom salts or use a different oil instead of almond.

Ingredients:

- 1 cup baking soda
- 1 cup citric acid
- ½ cup corn starch
- ½ cup of almond oil
- 5 to 8 drops jasmine essential oil (if using a fragrance oil use more drops to get the same scent and reduce the amount of water used)
- Pink food coloring (optional)

Method:

1. In a large glass bowl, mix the baking soda, corn starch, and citric acid until well combined with no clumps
2. Add the almond oil and essential oil, mixing well so it is evenly dispersed
3. Spray with water as required until the right consistency is achieved
4. Press firmly into molds (or shape by hand), leaving for a few hours before turning out on to wax paper and leaving overnight to dry

Orange Zesty Boost

I love oranges and find their scent very uplifting and refreshing, which is captured in this bath bomb. Feel free to add some body glitter if you really want to sparkle when you come out of the bath!

Ingredients:
- 1 cup baking soda
- ½ cup corn starch
- ½ cup citric acid
- ¼ cup Epsom salts
- 2 tablespoons almond oil
- 1 tablespoon water
- ½ teaspoon orange essential oil
- Orange food coloring

Method:
1. Put the dry ingredients into a large glass bowl and mix well, breaking up any clumps
2. In a separate bowl, whisk together the wet ingredients
3. Combine the two sets of ingredients and mix very well (add the glitter now if you are using it)
4. Spray with water, if required, until the correct consistency is achieved
5. Press firmly into your molds, leaving for an hour or two before turning out on to wax paper to dry overnight

Peppermint & Rosemary Wakeup

Another two of my favorite scents which are particular invigorating when combined, making it great after a hard gym session or to wake you up in the morning!

Ingredients:
- 1½ cups baking soda
- ½ cup Epsom salts
- ½ cup citric acid
- 1½ tablespoons almond oil
- ¼ teaspoon each of peppermint and rosemary essential oils
- Few drops of green food coloring

Method:
1. Mix the dry ingredients together in a large glass bowl, breaking up any lumps, until well combined
2. Stir in the wet ingredients, ensuring they are evenly dispersed
3. Spray with water, if required, until the correct consistency is achieved
4. Press firmly into molds, removing after a couple of hours and leaving to dry on wax paper overnight

Luxury Lavender Melt

After a hard day there is nothing quite like lavender to help you relax and let go of the stress. This bath bomb is perfect to release the week's stresses, so you can enjoy your weekend. Make it even more luxurious by pressing some dried lavender flowers or leaves (or both) into the mold before adding the bath bomb mixture.

Ingredients:
- 1 cup baking soda
- 2/3 cup citric acid
- 2/3 cup sea salt
- 2/3 cup cocoa butter (melted)
- 1/3 cup ground oatmeal
- 1/3 cup sodium lauryl sulfoacetate
- Lavender, lemon or peppermint essential oils
- Purple food coloring

Method:
1. Mix the dry ingredients together in a large glass bowl until well combined, breaking up any clumps (you may want to wear gloves and a mask with the sodium lauryl sulfoacetate as in powdered form it can become airborne and irritate your lungs – don't worry though, it is safe in the bath bomb)
2. In a separate bowl, mix together the cocoa butter and essential oils – use a few drops of each until you get a scent combination you like – I use 10 drops lavender and five drops of lemon though I have found 10 drops of peppermint and 5 drops of lemon to be particularly nice, giving it a mint chocolate smell!
3. Add the wet ingredients to the dry, including any food coloring, and stir well until event dispersed
4. Spray with water, if required, until the correct consistency is achieved
5. Pack the mixture firmly into a mold (a cake tin, jello mold or cupcake pan works well here) and leave in your refrigerator for about an hour to harden
6. Turn it out on to wax paper, leave overnight to dry, then cut into bars

ENDNOTE

Making your own bath bombs is surprisingly easy once you get used to getting the right consistency. It also works out cheaper than buying your own, particularly the expensive hand-made ones and can be turned into a very profitable business or just a source of a bit of extra money.

You can really let your artistic side loose when making bath bombs, both in the design, the coloring, and even the packaging with people prepared to pay a premium price for good quality, good looking bath bombs. They have become incredibly popular and sell well at craft fairs, farmer's markets and many other events.

You can even create your own website and sell online through that or through online auction and selling sites. This is a good way of creating some extra money to supplement your income, just remember to complete any required tax return information at the end of each year.

For me though, one of the biggest benefits is being able to make the bath bomb I want, meaning I can use the oils and other ingredients my skin needs. For anyone who suffers from allergies, this is ideal as you have complete control over the ingredients and know that what you are making is safe for you. If you have any skin problems you can use the information in this book to formulate bath bombs that can help ease those skin problems, which is a huge benefit for you.

It is great to be able to give someone who you know struggles to find beauty products they can use, something that they can enjoy and use without worrying that it will make their skin flare up. There is a surprisingly vibrant market for products such as these because few big manufacturers make suitable bath bombs.

Enjoy making your own bath bombs. Most of what you need you can find locally, though it is often easier to order online and have everything you need sent to your door. It's a big time saver and often works out much cheaper, particularly if you are buying in bulk. Some of the key items are more expensive than you think when bought from a supermarket compared to buying in bulk. I recently bought a lot of baking soda from a wholesaler and ended up paying the same for a kilo of it as I would have paid for a small tub of it from a supermarket. It is definitely worth shopping around, remember that if you are wanting to make money from this, you need to keep your costs low in order to maximize your profits.

Have fun with this process and enjoy the resulting bath bombs … you can relax and enjoy a wonderful bath knowing that you are testing your handiwork, so can spend as long as you want in there!

If you have enjoyed this book, please leave a review on Amazon as I love to hear from my readers and their successes with these methods.

Other Books by Jenny

Please check out my other health, cooking and beauty books on Amazon, available on Kindle and paperback. Get these books for free on Kindle Unlimited as part of your Amazon Prime membership.

Beauty

Home-Made Body Lotions - 30 Organic Body Lotion Recipes for Amazing Skin

Find out how you can make your own completely natural and healthy skin moisturizers at home. Whether you like creams, body butters or lotions, there are recipes galore in here as you learn how to make creams that treat dry skin, acne, oily skin, sensitive skin, normal skin and more including some special treats that also make great gifts!

Cooking

50 Meatball Recipes to Die For

Over 50 different meatball recipes that are mouth-wateringly delicious! Whether you like turkey, beef, pork or lamb meatballs you will find recipe after recipe here to impress your friends, win a cook-off or just enjoy a good meal. With sauce recipes too there is something here for everyone and you'll find this book packed full of recipes you can't wait to try!

99 Delicious Smoothie Recipes for A Healthier, Thinner You

Smoothies are a wonderful way to benefit from the vitamins, minerals and health boost from fruits and vegetables plus they are fantastic for anyone who is slimming. With 99 delicious recipes in this book you will be spoilt for choice and can find some great recipes you will love and enjoy!

Cooking With Coffee - 40 Delicious Coffee Recipes For The Coffee Lover

Coffee is one of the most under-used and under-stated ingredients in cookery yet it makes for delicious desserts and mouth-watering main courses, locking in the flavor and giving a dish a rich, full taste. Find out why coffee is so good for you and how you can use it to make the tastiest meals ever with over 40 main courses, desserts and drinks that will blow your taste buds!

The Mediterranean Diet Cookbook - 100 Delicious Yet Healthy Mediterranean Diet Recipes

Proven to be probably the healthiest diet on the planet, the Mediterranean diet is one that promotes good health, long life and vitality! Discover the secrets of the Mediterranean people and how the food they eat benefits their health. Learn why the Western diet is so unhealthy and find out how you can enjoy these delicious and healthy recipes which will improve your health and help you to lose weight.

Health

The Coconut Oil Miracle - Health Benefits, Weight Loss, Recipes and More

Coconut oil is being hailed as a miracle oil as Western society wakes up to this incredible oil that has potent benefits for your health, beauty, hair, skin and more! Find out all about this incredible oil and how it can benefit your health and help you feel fantastic. Includes over 40 delicious recipes, health tips, beauty tips and more!

ABOUT THE AUTHOR

Jenny De Luca is passionate about health and well-being, investing her time in learning to cook health improving meals and discovering natural and safe beauty products. She continues to learn more about how eating healthy food can significantly reduce the risk of chronic illness and combat many of the problems Western society faces today.

Made in United States
Troutdale, OR
09/24/2023

13155378R00046